Understanding Dementia and Caregiving for Your Aging Parents From A to Z

ISBN: 978-1484148297

Gerst, Ellen
Understanding Dementia and Caregiving
for Your Aging Parents From A to Z

Understanding Dementia and Caregiving for Your Aging Parents From A to Z

Ellen Gerst

TABLE OF CONTENTS

INTRODUCTION

In this age of information, if your loved one has been diagnosed with dementia, of which Alzheimer's is the most common type, you may rush to research all there is to know about the disease.

Since human beings are natural seekers, in an attempt to bring order to their world and to understand it better, they look for a cause and effect. Consequently, you hope that, if you understand dementia and its ramifications, you can come to understand the best ways to deal with its effects.

I *do* believe that understanding will give you a base of knowledge upon which to build, and this helps you to feel that you have some control over the situation. However, information alone, or beyond a certain point, isn't the only ingredient you will need in order to cope with a dementia diagnosis.

In truth, you are about to jump onto a rollercoaster of emotion, as you travel with your loved ones on a journey that will be fraught with lots of confusion, frustration, and unknowns.

This book is *not* an attempt to educate you on all the medical aspects of dementia, although I do touch on it gently. Instead, it speaks to you from the heart and a personal standpoint. It lets you know some of what to expect, and the emotions and thoughts you might have in response to your loved one's deteriorating condition.

Most of all, this book was written to share a journey upon which I am traveling with one of my loved ones, from the first recognition that something was awry to the hard decisions that needed to be made to ensure her safety and proper care.

While each person travels a unique road, many experience universal underlying truths and emotions about caring for aging loved ones, especially those afflicted with disease. When these truths are shared, caregivers are able to validate their own feelings, as well as alleviate some of the natural fearful and isolating thoughts they may have.

According to Julius Caesar, "experience is the teacher of all things." In view of that, I ask you to grab hold of my hand, and let me lend you support born from my experience.

I always like to imagine that if we all outstretched our hands to help the next person starting on this journey, soon, the whole world could be holding hands and supporting each other as they walk the treacherous and scary roads of dementia and caregiving.

In the following pages, with a focus on dementia of an Alzheimer's type, I share with you a compendium of twenty-six words and explanations, from A to Z, that I feel best express and validate what you are about to experience as you begin caregiving for your aging parents or another loved one.

UNDERSTANDING FROM A TO Z

*"Become aware that there are no accidents
in our intelligent universe.*

*Realize that everything that shows up in your life
has something to teach you.*

Appreciate everyone and everything in your life."

~Wayne Dyer

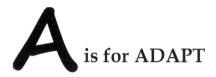 is for ADAPT

♦ADAPT: to make fit, often by modification

As you age, especially after the age of fifty, there are many adjustments you must make. Your mind tells you that you can stay up late and get up early; work all day and play at night; or simply jump up out of bed and be raring to go. However, your body says, *"Whoa, Nellie!"*

Your bones are creakier, your joints less elastic, and your energy level might be waning. You might also be noticing a little bit of forgetfulness, and the correct word or the idea you wished to express seems to vanish from your train of thought. Your eyesight is no longer 20/20, and you're turning up the volume on the television a notch so you can hear it better. These are all normal and gradual signs of gentle aging. They are manageable, and you learn to adapt to your *new normal* in order to continue to live a full life.

Now, multiply these new behaviors by ten or more and the picture you draw is of your aging parents who are no longer able to complete tasks by themselves.

Just when you thought you were home free to enjoy your long awaited retirement, your parents need your help. A role reversal takes place, for with increasing frailty of both body and mind, your parents, in essence, become your children. However, these aren't children who are managed easily.

After all, your parents are adults and have most likely led independent lives up until now. It is a very big adjustment for them to relinquish their adult freedoms, even if it is for their own safety.

There will be a period of upheaval and transition while both you and your parents become accustomed and adapt to these new circumstances and the rules that come with it.

"When we are no longer able to change a situation, we are challenged to change ourselves."

~Victor Frankl

"Life is neither static nor unchanging. With no individuality, there can be no change, no adaption and, in an inherently changing world, any species unable to adapt is also doomed."

~Jean M. Auel

B is for BRAIN FUNCTION

♦ BRAIN FUNCTION: how the healthy and non-healthy brain works

Despite weighing only three pounds, the brain contains more than 100 billion cells, including neurons (nerve cells) that send signals to thousands of other cells at the rate of 200 miles per hour. It is your most vital organ and is responsible for keeping you functioning. It manages your involuntary life support systems, as well as determining your personality and keeping your memory functional.

Starting at age 20 and continuing through age 90, the brain loses five to ten percent of its weight. Originally, it was theorized that from birth onward neurons were lost naturally, and this was part of the shrinking process and a cause of age-related memory loss. Subsequently, it was discovered that neurons have the ability to remain healthy in the absence of a specific disease that causes neuron death.

Aging also causes the grooves on the surface of the brain to widen, while the swellings on the surface become smaller. Additionally, there is an increase in the decay of the branch-like fingers (dendrites) that extend from the neurons. Over time, senile plaques, which are hard clusters of these damaged and decaying neurons, start to form and cut off some of the messaging capability of the brain.

One of the distinguishing features of Alzheimer's Disease (AD) is the accumulation of amyloid plaques between the neurons in the brain. The body naturally produces amyloids, which are protein fragments. A healthy brain is able to eliminate these fragments, while in a brain affected by AD, the fragments accumulate and harden to form insoluble plaques. These amyloids tend to form in the area of the brain that is responsible for forming new memories and interferes with the brain's mechanism of long-term memory. In addition to being associated with AD, amyloids play a role in many other neurodegenerative disorders such as Huntington's Disease, Parkinson's, and Diabetes Type 2.

Researchers believe that at the heart of plaque formation is a chemical reaction that inflames the brain. A decline in dopamine is another chemical process that affects brain aging. Dopamine is the brain chemical associated with pleasure and reward. With the steady loss of this chemical, the metabolism in the region of the brain related to cognition slows down.

More recent studies are now postulating that amyloids are actually secreted by the brain to defend itself against a new culprit, tau protein, which is being branded as an infection of sorts. Tau proteins are found in abundance in the neurons of the central nervous system. When these proteins become defective, or are no longer able to do their job of stabilizing the body processes with which they are associated, the result can initiate the development of dementia of an Alzheimer's type.

Taking all this research into consideration, you might wonder if there are any preventative measures you can take in order to slow the onset of the ramifications of aging.

There *is* good news! Research indicates that the rate of brain aging can be hastened or slowed by lifestyle factors. Accordingly, some preventative measures you can take include the following.

1. Keep your blood glucose levels low to deter the production of inflammatory proteins that can lead to the production of plaque.

2. Adhere to the *"use it or lose it"* principle and keep your brain active and challenged.

3. Exercise, which could mean as little as walking rapidly for a minimum of 45 minutes, three times a week.

4. Establish a regular pattern of eight hours of sleep per night.

5. Keep stress in check to decrease the overproduction of cortisol.

6. Watch your diet to keep hypertension in check because medicine for this condition can accelerate aging and shrink the brain.

"The human brain, then, is the most complicated organization of matter that we know."

~Issac Asimov

C is for COUNSELING

♦ COUNSELING: treatment for psychological issues

Your parents are acting out of character. They may have become more argumentative, belligerent or paranoid. You attempt to have a rational conversation with them and try to get to the bottom of their complaints and new attitude. There seems to be a lack of a good explanation. You may think to yourself, *"Are my parents crazy or am I?"* It turns out that neither of you are crazy. Changes such as these may indicate the beginning of a demented state or another medical issue that gives rise to a disruption in normal behavioral patterns.

As a rule of thumb, if your parents are having psychological problems, an insurance-covered visit to a therapist may be indicated. The good news is that Medicare will not only cover visits to a therapist for your parents but for you as the caregiver as well. It is in a therapeutic setting that you can learn what to expect and how to address issues as your parents move through the stages of dementia. You can also explore your feelings and validate your own sanity.

It is natural to be emotional about your parents' condition, and you will most likely experience the highs and lows that come with this event. However, if you are going to be caregiving on an everyday basis, it will be difficult to exist in a state of constant high emotion and still retain your own equilibrium.

Although to an outsider it may seem a bit harsh, approaching your parents' care with a more clinical attitude may be your saving grace.

Adopting this method doesn't mean that you have stopped loving your parents. *This is very far from the truth.* By embracing this type of attitude, you are better able to deal with the hard decisions to be made and the aberrant behavior that may be exhibited. It would be very difficult for you to function well in your own life, if you constantly let your emotions be in charge.

As with everything, there is a proper time and place to feel your emotions and a time to keep them in check.

"Don't let mental blocks control you.
Set yourself free.
Confront your fear and
turn the mental blocks into building blocks."

~Roopleen, Words To Inspire The Winner in YOU

"To give vent now and then to his feelings,
whether of pleasure or discontent,
is a great ease to a man's heart."

~Francesco Guicciardini

D is for DEMENTIA

♦ **DEMENTIA: the gradual deterioration of mental functioning, which affects a person's ability to perform normal daily activities**

Many use the terms Alzheimer's and dementia interchangeably, as I also do throughout this book. However, dementia is actually a *symptom* caused by Alzheimer's Disease (AD). To understand the difference, a good analogy is that an elevated temperature is not a disease, but rather a *symptom* of some underlying malady that causes a spike in temperature.

When dementia is present, a person exhibits significant memory problems along with other cognitive disabilities that interfere with the completion of the everyday tasks of life.

This does not happen overnight. In fact, the walk towards a demented state is a slow and progressive one. The earliest and telltale signs can include: memory loss, confusion, changes in behavior, and communication difficulties. As the underlying disease of the dementia develops, the patient can experience difficulty with problem solving, understanding new concepts, learning new skills, and decision making. Changes in personality may also occur and can include an increase of incidences of fear, anger, and paranoia, as well as depressive symptoms.

If you begin to notice similar symptoms or other behavioral changes in your parents, it's important to solicit a proper diagnosis from a licensed specialist who will administer various tests to determine the cause and its severity. Even a specialist, though, can only make a presumption of the presence of AD because a definitive diagnosis can't be made while a person is alive.

Although AD is at the root of most cases of dementia (70-80%), there are other dementia causing diseases that have distinct symptom patterns of which to be aware. Moreover, old age is not the only cause of dementia. It can be brought on by a variety of circumstances, including a high fever, dehydration, Lyme disease, long term substance abuse, poor nutrition or a brain tumor.

Vascular Dementia is the second most common type and is caused by a decreased blood flow to parts of the brain. This is most often caused by a series of small strokes that block arteries.

Dementia with Lewy Bodies is diagnosed when there are abnormal deposits of Lewy bodies, or the protein alphasynuclein, inside the nerve cells of the brain. Along with AD-like symptoms, there may be visual hallucinations, muscle rigidity and tremors.

Normal Pressure Hydrocephalus occurs when there is buildup of fluid in the brain. This can sometimes be alleviated with surgery and the installation of a brain shunt to drain the excess fluid.

Mild Cognitive Impairment is diagnosed when a person experiences memory issues and has some cognitive dysfunction, but they are not severe enough to interfere with the daily tasks of life. This condition can progress to full blown dementia or remain constant.

Frontotemporal Dementia is diagnosed when damage to the brain cells is found, especially in the front and side areas. Typically, a change in personality and behavior, along with language difficulties, is observed.

Mixed Dementia is diagnosed when one or more types of dementia are indicated, usually Alzheimer's and vascular, but can include some of the others too.

Parkinson's Disease is often a precursor to the development of dementia and occurs in the later stages of the disease.

Creuzfeldt-Jakob Disease is thought to be caused by eating cattle affected with Mad Cow Disease. This variation of dementia progresses rapidly, causing memory and coordination impairment and behavioral changes.

"I often hear people say that a person suffering from Alzheimer's is not the person they knew.
I wonder to myself, *Who are they now?*"

~Bob DeMarco, The Alzheimer's Reading Room
www.alzheimersreadingroom.com

E is for ENERGY LEVEL

◆ **ENERGY LEVEL: a stable state of constant energy that may be assumed by a physical system**

A night of refreshing sleep can sharpen your cognitive ability as well as increase your energy level. Unfortunately, many elders experience sleep disturbances that affect their ability to optimally function during the day. They can experience difficulty falling or staying asleep; early morning awakening; or excessive daytime sleepiness. Contributing factors to these disturbances can include: physical maladies (chronic or acute); medication side effects; psychiatric disorders; and interruptions in routines and other social changes.

It's a tough decision for a doctor to prescribe sleep inducing medication, for sedation can lead to increased disorientation, which can be at the root of more accidents and falls. Before deciding to administer any remedy, over-the-counter or otherwise, much discussion is required with your parents' team of medical professionals.

Interrupted sleep, combined with your parents' advanced age, is a prescription for a slowdown of activity. If your parents live in a community that offers activities, which even you find intriguing, you may strongly encourage them to participate. If they decline, you may get upset, asking *"Why don't you want to attend these activities? Isn't it better than just staying in your apartment every day?"*

What you might have to realize (and accept) is that your parents may not have the strength, the attention span, or even the ability to concentrate for a long enough period of time that would allow them to meaningfully participate in cultural or social activities.

Furthermore, after a lifetime of similar activities, perhaps their attitude is *"been there, done that"* and they don't want to listen to lectures, see a movie or play bingo.

While at times it may seem as if your parents are your children, they are *not* and you need to learn to respect their wishes. They have lost so much freedom; let them decide for themselves whether they have enough energy or desire to participate in their community's offerings.

**"Without enough sleep,
We all become tall two-year olds."**

*~JoJo Jensen,
Dirt Famer Wisdom, 2002*

**"Nobody realizes that some people
expend tremendous energy merely to be normal."**

~Albert Camus

F is for FAMILY UNITY

♦ **FAMILY UNITY: a lack of discordance between family members; ability to agree and trust**

Often, one child bears more of the burden of caring for elderly parents than his or her siblings. It may be a question of geography, finances or temperament. Whatever the reason, the person who is in the trenches dealing with all the issues that arise each day needs the full support of the other family members.

When tending to aging parents, especially those exhibiting dementia or dementia-like qualities, frustration is sure to arise. Caregivers need to have *someone* available to them, ideally a sibling or another close family member, with whom they can vent and express their feelings *sans* judgment.

In general, you can talk to close family members about your parents, even with anger, and they will know your comments don't negate the love you hold for them; hence, there is no judgment. However, when you speak to an *outsider*, it may be a different situation.

Rather than driving caregivers to suppress the types of emotion which can be detrimental to their physical and mental health, *or* to be forced to look outside the family for someone in whom to confide who may not be as understanding, be the shoulder upon which they can vent and cry. Listen with a loving heart and an open ear.

Most often, caregivers are simply looking for catharsis, rather than asking you for solutions to problems for which there are none. Listening in silence may be the right kind of support that is needed to lighten their load.

As an addendum, this also precludes caregivers from burdening a spouse with tales of frustration about parental behavior. In this way, you may be saving a marriage, too.

**"The most basic and powerful way to connect
to another person is to listen. Just listen.**

**A loving silence often has far more power to heal and
to connect than most well-intentioned words."**

~Rachel Naomi Remen

**Don't say to the sibling who is acting as
the main parental caregiver,
*"You're so strong. I couldn't do what you do."***

You may *think* you're offering a compliment, but this is NOT a helpful comment. It also may be indicative of the fact that you really don't know your sibling at all.

While the caregiver may outwardly be *acting with strength*, she feels anything but strong inside. In fact, she may be dying a thousand little deaths each time a parent's condition deteriorates right in front of her eyes. However, she has been given no choice (*often by the abdication of her siblings*) but to simply do what needs to be done. *And, so she does.*

G is for GLASS HALF FULL

♦ GLASS HALF FULL: a way of viewing circumstances from a positive vantage point

You have probably heard a variation of the story that tells of two people who look at the same situation and one sees the glass half full and the other half empty. It comes down to a matter of perspective.

In truth, every event in life is neutral. It is the individual who will color it with emotion in order to categorize and label the "event" as a positive or a negative one.

Please do not misunderstand this statement.

This does *not* mean you should ignore or deny your feelings. It's natural for you to be upset and emotional that your parents are aging, frail or suffering from dementia-like symptoms and not able to care for themselves. What is neutral about the event is that, while it's true, you can't change the facts about the situation – even though you wish you could.

Where your power lies now is in how you will ultimately *reflectively respond* vs. *reflexively react* to your parents' situation.

You will also have to decide the size of the role which you will play in their lives going forward and contemplate the effect of that decision on your life, as well as on your conscience.

As you come to grips with their mortality and your own, rather than denying your feelings, you need to fully embrace your emotions because that is how you will process them through your body. Part of your emotional work may also include pre-grieving the loss of the parents who once cared for you as you now switch roles.

"For myself, I am an optimist.
It does not seem to be much use being anything else."

~*Sir Winston Churchill*

"One's suffering disappears when one lets oneself go,
when one yields – even to sadness."

~*Antoine de Saint-Exupéry*

"How much has to be explored and discarded
before reaching the naked flesh of feeling?"

~*Claude Debussy*

H is for HONESTY

♦ HONESTY: strict adherence to the facts

If one or both of your parents are exhibiting dementia-like symptoms or have been diagnosed with another serious disease, you are faced with the dilemma of whether to share this news with them. At times, total honesty may *not* be the best policy.

Of course, you would rather be upfront and tell the truth. However, as you ponder your decision, ask yourself what purpose it would fulfill to tell them of a difficult diagnosis. Would your parents be better served, or even understand the ramifications of a dementia diagnosis, *or* do you want to tell them because of your own frustration with their new behaviors and your sadness about the situation?

The word Alzheimer's strikes fear in the heart and mind of every baby boomer.

Each time you misplace your keys, can't remember what's on your shopping list or someone's name, you might secretly question yourself, *"Am I heading towards Alzheimer's?"*

The answer is probably not. Gradual memory loss is a natural sign of aging. Alzheimer's is marked with a much deeper type of memory loss and the breakdown of the ability to reason logically.

Therefore, even if you explain to your parents that they have Alzheimer's, and that is why they are having trouble remembering or believe someone is taking their things, it will be virtually impossible for them to grasp your logical explanation. The usual result is frustration on everyone's part, and it's possible that your parents may become more agitated and frightened by what is to come.

Deep reflection, including a careful evaluation of the result you hope to achieve by informing your parents of their infirmity, is warranted. After weighing the medical community's advice, it is a personal decision based on what you think would be in your parents' best interest vs. your best interest.

I ask you to consider the idea that it's possible to still tell the truth without naming the truth. For example, you can talk about the ramifications of memory issues without mentioning the term Alzheimer's.

"The truth is more important than the facts."

~Frank Lloyd Wright

I is for INDEPENDENT LIVING CENTER

♦ INDEPENDENT LIVING: a living arrangement that can alleviate the burden of home ownership

Life is a series of revisions – in your attitudes, your living arrangements, your familial structure and a host of others areas.

When aging parents can no longer live in their own home due to extensive upkeep and maintenance, there are decisions to be made which will play a big part in their quality of life. There is a tiered hierarchy of options available, which includes independent living to assisted living to a nursing home. The choice depends on both the physical and mental health of your parents.

In general, independent living facilities are senior communities that cater to those 55 years and older. The choices are wide reaching and range from apartment living *to* free standing homes (which have low to no maintenance) *to* specialized facilities that offer meals, transportation and cleaning services, and appropriately geared activities.

Depending on the funds available, there are various options available that include, but are not limited to, the following.

1. *Subsidized senior housing*, which often has a very long waiting list

2. *Senior apartments*, which are age-restricted and may include services such as transportation, meals, cleaning and activities

3. *Retirement communities*, which are age-restricted and consist of different types of housing units, ranging from single family homes to condos

4. *Continuing care retirement communities*, which offer packages that allow access to independent living, assisted living and skilled nursing care with transfers allowed between them as needed

"Changes that make life
more satisfying don't occur overnight.
But, for people who are *willing to work*
toward greater independence, independent living
centers can help put the pieces together."

~*ILRU at Texas Institute for Rehabilitation*

J is for JOURNAL WRITING

♦ JOURNAL WRITING: periodic entries of feelings and chronicling of life events *plus* your reaction to them

Putting pen to paper and producing the written word is a magical medium that allows your thoughts to flow smoothly from you to another person. There's no body language to confuse the listener or a chance to misconstrue a tone of voice. In essence, it is a vehicle that allows you to communicate without being present.

A journal can serve various purposes. It may simply be a private memo to yourself. Although, if you so desire, your thoughts may also be read by the masses *or* by the one special person to whom they are directed. Some of these factors can allow you to be more comfortable to fearlessly express your emotions *vs.* feeling hesitant if you were to try to convey them in an oral format.

Journal writing is especially helpful when you find yourself in a negative frame of mind, for example, when you are frustrated with parents who are increasingly frail and headed toward or are in a demented state.

By recording the adverse feelings you may be experiencing, you are actually releasing them from your body and staving off possible harmful physical effects. Take note that it's also important to chronicle moments of happiness and joy, so your journal doesn't turn into a diatribe of despair.

It is also a good idea to periodically review your journal entries, especially when you are having a hard day. When your journal is a compilation of both your positive and negative thoughts, upon review, you can see that your life is neither good nor bad, but a balance of the two. It can also illustrate the progress you're making in accepting your parents' fate.

"Fill your paper with the breathings of your heart."

~William Wordsworth

**"The act of putting pen to paper
encourages pause for thought.
In turn, this makes us think more deeply about life,
which helps us regain our equilibrium."**

~Norbett Platt

K is for KNOWLEDGE *vs.* EMOTION

♦ **KNOWLEDGE *vs.* EMOTION: practical information lacking emotional input is not a complete picture**

If your parents have received a *Dementia of an Alzheimer's type* diagnosis, or if they are simply becoming frailer in their old age, you have probably researched future options in regard to living arrangements and medical care. Although this is a terrific start, sometimes "book" knowledge is not enough for you to come to terms with your particular situation.

Family, and parents in particular, lies at the foundation of your stability. Despite your independence, or the many miles you may live from your parents, it's still comforting to know that they are accessible for advice, comfort and support.

No matter what age you are, when your parents die, you will consider yourself an orphan. Without parents, it makes you one of the elder statespersons of your family. In the normal scheme of things, this makes you "next up."

This thought may be rumbling around in your mind, tucked very far away so that you don't have to think about it. However, your unconscious mind is aware of these musings, and it can make you uneasy, which is a natural state of being as you face your own mortality.

There are many options to help you adjust to the new roles you will be playing, including therapy and support groups for children of AD patients.

Although each familial situation is unique, there are many universal truths that can be revealed in the safe environment of a support group.

Each person tells his story, and as you touch the lives of others and they reciprocate, you initiate the healing process. This is also a place where your feelings are validated, and you learn you aren't alone in them. Additionally, you can gain perspective as you listen to those who are further along in their journey, as well as evaluate your own progress in coming to terms with your situation and that of your parents.

"The tragic or the humorous
is a matter of perspective."

~Arnold Beisser

"When dealing with people, remember
you are *not* dealing with creatures of logic,
but creatures of emotion."

~Dale Carnegie

"Your intellect may be confused,
but your emotions will never lie to you."

~Roger Ebert

L is for LOSS of FREEDOM

♦ LOSS of FREEDOM: the presence of necessity, coercion or constraint in choice or action

There are two aspects to the loss of freedom.

Your parents, as they move from independent living to some type of dependent living, experience diminishing freedom in return for abdicating most of their daily living responsibilities.

On the other end of the spectrum, the caregiver also experiences a loss of freedom and flexibility. To compensate, innovative methods must be developed in order to complete necessary personal and familial tasks in an efficient manner.

Both you and your parents might rebel against the new restraints placed in your life and be angry or act out in other ways. Because grief is a confusing emotion that manifests in many ways, you may not recognize that you and your parents are commencing the mourning process for the lives you once lived.

Your parents realize they are close to the end of their lives and that a move to some sort of facility is a move to the place where they will most likely die. On the other hand, you feel both constrained and, perhaps, guilty that you resent these constraints.

As a loving, responsible child, you attempt to bury these feelings and complete the necessary tasks with a smile. *Unfortunately*, ignoring your feelings won't make them go away; they only fester to later explode and create havoc.

 Many who mourn do the same, for society hasn't taught its members how to deal with loss in a healthy manner. And loss, *in any form*, must be understood and accepted before figuring out how to move forward.

Let go of guilt; it's a useless emotion. Accept that it's natural for you to war with your conscience – to feel obligated to help because you love your parents, yet resentful that it interferes with your own enjoyment.

Knowing and accepting that you *can't* and *won't* desert your parents in their time of need, it becomes your job to develop systems and a network of support to allow you to balance your own needs with those of your aging parents.

**"Guilt:
the gift that keeps on giving."**

~Erma Bombeck

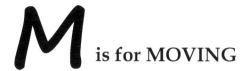 **is for MOVING**

♦ MOVING: to change locations

No matter how old you are, change is difficult and uncomfortable, even if it means a situation will get better. For the older population, any sort of change in their normal routine magnifies this effect.

While a younger person can go with the flow, for example, adjusting to a new home, for an older person, moving can be a defining event that heralds the onset of confusion.

Remain aware of this fact, especially if your parents have lived independently in a part of the country far from you, and you decide that now it would be prudent to have them move closer to your city or state. When a person has lived in one home or one city for numerous years, the patterns of life become ingrained in the brain and tasks are completed by rote. When a new living environment is introduced in a new city, or even in a different area of the same city, life becomes more difficult and bewildering.

Your parents may not remember that they downsized and that you disposed of old or broken pieces in order for their important possessions to fit in smaller quarters. They insist that items they owned thirty years ago are being stolen; they can't figure out and remember how new appliances work – no matter how many times you explain it to them; or they may wander off and get lost.

They are not trying to be difficult; it is that they have been robbed of their ability to remember and reason with logic. Moreover, keep in mind that at a later stage in life, most people are hard-pressed to make new information and patterns stick.

Additionally, if your parents don't live in the same city or state as you, it may be hard to determine what is true or false. If you are receiving an increasing amount of panicked phone calls about things that are missing or that "someone" is stealing their things, this could be an initial tipoff for you to further investigate their ability to live independently and far from familial help.

**"All change is not growth,
as all movement is not forward."**

~Ellen Glasgow

**"There are lots of people who mistake
their imagination for their memory."**

~Josh Billings

**"Memory is a complicated thing,
a relative to truth, but not its twin."**

~Barbara Kingsolver, Animal Dreams

N is for NURSING HOME *vs.* ASSISTED LIVING

♦ NURSING HOME: living arrangement with 24/7 skilled nursing care available

♦ ASSISTED LIVING: living arrangement for those who need moderate assistance with daily living tasks

Although it's possible to care for an aging parent at home, with or without dementia symptoms, eventually the burden may become too great. Consequently, some sort of outside or additional care may be necessary. The options range from adult day services *to* assisted living *to* respite or nursing home care. There are also facilities that cater specifically to dementia patients called memory care units.

Adult Day Services or Elder Care Programs. These provide activities for adults who need assistance. They usually operate during daytime and weekday hours only and may include lunch and transportation to and from the facility. There are programs that are specifically designed for AD patients, but other programs exist for those who are mentally capable but have physical ailments that make it difficult to complete activities on their own.

Home Health Services. There are many companies who cater to assisting the elderly with personal care such as meal preparation and eating, taking medications, bathing, dressing, and grooming. Some agencies can provide a caregiver to run errands or help with household chores. Additional specialized services are also available, such as wound care and physical therapy.

Respite Care. This type of care caters more to the caregiver *vs.* the care receiver. When a caregiver is tied down at home, the daily chores of life become more difficult to complete. Some community organizations or even friends, good neighbors and family members can provide a needed break for caregivers to regroup, refresh and rejuvenate.

Nursing Home. If your parents are in need of daily medical attention, a nursing home may be your best option. Twenty-four hour nursing care is provided, along with socialization activities, room and board. There are nursing homes that have specialized units for Alzheimer's patients.

Assisted Living. This type of arrangement works best for those people who have moderate functional impairment but can essentially care for themselves with some assistance. Everyday medical care is not necessary, and they can navigate their own living quarters. Most often, laundry and cleaning services, activities, and personal care assistance with bathing and dressing are available, as well as dining room service for three meals.

Assisted living facilities can come in the form of a group home where each person has his or her own bedroom and meals are eaten collectively, or it can be a larger facility where each person has his or her own living quarters. In the case of the latter, there is also a communal dining room and lounge areas where planned activities take place. The living quarters are very often the size of a large hospital room or a studio apartment. A private bathroom is attached to the room, and usually a microwave and small refrigerator are included. Bedroom furniture, a comfortable chair or a very small loveseat, and, possibly, a small kitchen table can fit in the room.

Memory Care Units. These are designed especially for dementia patients. There is a more institutionalized feel about this type of facility, and they are usually on the smaller size with, perhaps, 20 rooms available. Each person has a private unit, approximately 250 square feet. Residents are encouraged to bring their own furniture and special belongings to personalize the room, which can help to stir their memory. There are common areas such as a dining area, recreation area, beauty shop, and outside areas. There are also smaller facilities that may house only 4 to 6 people. A "regular" house is utilized and each person has his or her own bedroom.

Whichever level of care you choose for your parents, it is important to investigate each thoroughly. Ask for a recommendation from medical professionals. Take the time to tour different facilities. Interview staff members until you are comfortable with all the answers you receive.

"Most Americans have some experience with nursing homes or other long term care settings, and nearly half have had a family member or close friend in a home in the past three years."

~Michael Burgess

**"Be nice to your kids.
They'll choose your nursing home."**

~Anonymous

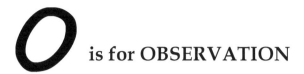

is for OBSERVATION

♦ OBSERVATION: a judgment on or inference from information collected

It is imperative to make regular reassessments of your parents' ability to live independently or to be left alone for any period of time.

Caregiving is a dynamic process that must adapt to the constant changes that your parents are experiencing. Some of these changes may be subtle, for example, your parents may only complain when you leave the house or don't come to visit them often enough.

While you try to rationally reason with them by saying that you'll only be gone for an hour or so, there may be an underlying emotion that is causing this behavior, such as fear. They may be cognizant enough to recognize their limited ability to react properly in an emergency or to deal with something unexpected. Consequently, something benign to you, such as the telephone ringing or someone knocking on the door, could provoke a frightened and agitated state.

To help you determine the level of attention and care your parents may need, the following are a few basic questions for which you need to determine the answers.

1. Will your parents "stay put" or wander off if left unattended? If so, do they know where they live and how to get back home?

2. In an emergency, do they understand how to leave the home (or an apartment building) if necessary?

3. Are they capable of any meal production, for example, one that doesn't require the use of an appliance that generates heat? Do they understand the danger of leaving a hot stove unattended?

4. Do they know how to access emergency services, for example, how to call 911 or how to use a personal call button?

5. If they were to have a life-threatening medical emergency that requires medication, are they able to administer it themselves, for example, a dose of nitroglycerin or a shot of insulin?

6. Are they capable of attending to bathroom rituals by themselves?

**"Observation –
an activity of both eyes and ears."**

~Horace Mann

**"To acquire knowledge, one must study;
But to acquire wisdom, one must observe."**

~Marilyn Vos Savant

P is for PARANOIA

♦ PARANOIA: tendency toward excessive *or* irrational suspiciousness *and* distrustfulness of others

Paranoia is a common symptom of dementia and often comes with criticism and personal attacks. Consequently, while you're trying your best to attend to the needs of your aging parents, you may also be dealing with accusations of lying and stealing or worse.

In order to move through these trying moments, it's important to avoid taking these attacks *personally*. These episodes aren't really about you; instead, they are a result of a combination of your parents' reduced capacity to reason and their failing memory. This is a prescription for utter exasperation.

No matter how times you explain the way monies were used or transferred to different bank accounts, parents may insist that it is missing and *you* must have stolen it.

What makes logical sense to you is gibberish to your parents, for the ability to apply logic to a situation has evaporated. In other words, if A = B and B = C, they can no longer make the leap that A = C.

Even if the logic of the situation does get through, with impaired short term memory, the explanation is soon forgotten and you find yourself repeating yourself ad nauseam.

It will be very difficult to convince your parents of your pure motives. However, *what you can do* is protect yourself against the accusations of other family members.

To avoid this situation, you might complete the following tasks.

1. Maintain detailed records of all funds and their usage.

2. Keep a written inventory with accompanying pictures of all possessions.

3. If possible, let your parents sign checks for prescribed expenses.

It is also imperative to protect yourself emotionally. You may want to speak to a therapist; confide in close friends or siblings; meditate in order to regain equilibrium; and acknowledge and accept that your accuser is simply the physical vessel of your parent and that it is a stranger who verbally attacks you. This can help to mitigate the enormous sting that a negative confrontation with a parent holds.

"Confusion is an often too subtle sign of paranoia."

~Anne Austin

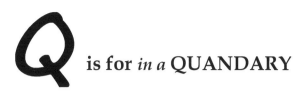 **is for** *in a* **QUANDARY**

♦ *in a* **QUANDARY: confused about how to proceed**

You might be noticing that your parents are acting out of character. If your parents live far away from you or your siblings, the concerned phone calls between you are flying fast and furious. If you're an only child, and/or perhaps single, you feel more alone as you have no one with whom to share your increasing concerns.

Typical questions you may ask yourself or your siblings include the following.

> *"What did Mom/Dad say to you? I heard a completely different story."*
>
> *"Do you think it's possible that someone is actually coming into their apartment and stealing things?"*
>
> *"Do you think it is safe for them to still drive?"*
>
> *"Do you think we need to consider moving them closer to one of us?"*
>
> *"Do you think they are taking their medications?"*
>
> *"Are you afraid that they'll forget to turn to oven off?"*

If you have not been exposed to anyone with Alzheimer's, you may not recognize some of these beginning stage symptoms. You're merely *in a quandary* and wondering what is causing this new turmoil in the lives of your up-until-now independent parents.

At first, you want to believe your parents that their possessions are missing or might have been stolen. You may become indignant for them and investigate the possibility of a robbery. When this situation arises repeatedly, and very often the items are eventually found, you begin to realize that there may be more going on than you originally thought.

This is the dawning of the recognition of a medical problem and that it's time for you to spring into action.

Although an Alzheimer's diagnosis is devastating, it can also bring you *some* piece of mind that there is a logical explanation for the changes you have observed in your parents' behavior.

"Perplexity is the beginning of knowledge."

~*Khalil Gibran*

R is for ROLL WITH THE PUNCHES

♦ ROLL WITH THE PUNCHES: able to deal with difficulties as they arise

Alzheimer's (AD) is a progressive disease. On a continuum, it may be quite manageable with only slight intervention required at the beginning stages, while, in the later stages, institutionalization with 24/7 care will probably be a necessity. Familiarizing yourself with the different stages of AD will allow you to successfully navigate and mitigate problems ahead of time that may endanger the lives of your parents as the disease advances, while, concurrently, trying your best to preserve their dignity and quality of life.

Dr. Barry Reisberg, *Clinical Director of the NYU School of Medicine's Silberstein Aging and Dementia Research Center*, states that AD is experienced in 7 stages, as follows, with the caveat that not everyone will experience the same symptoms or progress at the same rate.

1. *No impairment*. This is the base line and indicates normal function.

2. *Very mild cognitive decline*. This may only be normal age-related changes or the earliest signs of AD. There may be some memory lapse, but no other symptoms of dementia are noted.

3. *Mild cognitive decline*. Although difficult to diagnose definitively, this can be the onset of early-stage AD with symptoms including: difficulty with word finding; difficulty remembering new names and faces; greater difficulty performing social or work related tasks; losing or misplacing objects of value; increasing difficulty with planning or organizing; and forgetting material recently read.

4. *Moderate cognitive decline*. This is regarded as true mild or early-stage AD. A consultation with a neuro-psychologist who can administer testing for AD is indicated at this point. Areas to be examined include: frequency of forgetfulness of recent events; difficulty with challenging mental arithmetic, such as counting backwards from 100 by 7's; greater difficulty performing complex tasks such as managing finances; forgetfulness about one's life; and withdrawing from challenging social situations.

5. *Moderately severe cognitive decline*. Regarded as moderate or mid-stage AD, there are noticeable gaps in memory and thinking and help is needed to complete daily activities. Symptoms can include: the inability to recall own address and telephone number; confusion about the day of the week or physical location; difficulty with less challenging mental arithmetic, such as counting backwards from 20 by 2's; and help is needed to choose proper seasonal clothing. At this stage, significant details about themselves and their family are remembered, and there is no assistance required to eat or use the toilet.

6. *Severe cognitive decline*. Entering the moderately severe or (later) mid-stage AD, memory worsens; personality changes are observed; and extensive help is needed to complete daily activities. Symptoms may include: a loss of awareness of recent experiences; difficulty with personal history but still remembers own name; difficulty remembering the name of a spouse or caregiver; increasing help needed with daily tasks, such as dressing and toileting; lack of control of bladder or bowels; shifts in personality, including OCD symptoms and paranoia; and a tendency to wander or get lost.

7. *Very severe cognitive decline*. In this late-stage or final stage of AD, the following symptoms may be present: the inability to respond to the environment or to carry on a conversation, and, eventually, be unable to control movement. Muscles become rigid, which leads to an impairment in swallowing, smiling, and the ability to hold the head up. Help is needed to attend to personal care items such as eating and toileting. Communication is difficult with an eventual loss of word usage. Assistance is needed to walk with the eventual inability to do so. Vulnerability to infections, such as pneumonia, is also prevalent. This late-stage can last from several weeks to several years, and 24/7 help is usually required.

As you observe your parents, they may exhibit a symptom from one stage and others from a different stage. The preceding is simply a framework for you to study so that you can foster your ability to *"roll with the punches"* as each assault occurs on the minds and bodies of your parents.

S is for SUNDOWN SYNDROME

♦ **SUNDOWN SYNDROME: a condition most often associated with early-stage AD**

There is no clear definition of Sundown Syndrome. Instead, it's regarded as a phase that occurs during the time of transition between light and dark, either early in the morning or late in the afternoon. As the sun rises or wanes, you may notice that your parents exhibit increasing amounts of memory loss, confusion, anger and agitation. It's possible that hallucinations may be experienced, too, as the change in light creates shadows and plays havoc with deteriorating eyesight.

Be aware that dementia is not the only trigger for this syndrome. Otherwise healthy elders may also exhibit these symptoms after a surgery that included anesthesia, or they may start to occur during a long hospital stay.

Other triggers can include the following.

1. Fatigue

2. Lack of scheduled activities after dinner, which means less structure or routine

3. Shadowy or low light as mentioned above

4. Hormone imbalance or a misfiring internal clock that becomes more pronounced during the transition between waking and sleeping

5. Seasonal Affective Disorder (SAD), which is more prevalent in the short, dark days of winter

6. A change in shifts and personnel (if in a care facility)

Although there is no "cure" for Sundown Syndrome, there are ways to better manage the effects of it. It's important to remember that those suffering from dementia do best in a regimented routine with minimal changes or surprises. Establishing daily routines to be followed in the same way and at the same time can help keep your parents on an even keel.

The following six items are some other preventative procedures that you can implement in an attempt to provide more structure in your parents' environment.

1. Monitor their diet, especially watching caffeine and sugar intake

2. Keep noise to a minimum in the evening

3. Limit visitors that upset the established routine

4. Install a night light in the bedroom and bathroom

5. Explore light therapy to minimize SAD effects

6. Ask their doctor about medication that may help to minimize the effects of the syndrome

**"Monsters are real and ghosts are real, too.
They live inside of us, and sometimes they win."**
~Stephen King

T is for THIS COULD HAPPEN TO ME

♦ THIS COULD HAPPEN TO ME: concern for your own well-being

Alzheimer's Disease (AD) currently affects more than 5 million Americans, and it's the sixth leading killer in the U.S. Since the risk of developing AD increases with age, and our longevity is continually increasing, the number of people who will be affected is escalating exponentially. To counteract this upward trend, plans have been recently laid out by the federal government to have an effective treatment in place by 2025.

Does this mean that *you* need to be concerned about developing AD, especially if your parents have fallen victim to the disease? This thought is a natural and common one that can cause anxiety to build up as you question yourself every time you forget something.

Remember, though, a "normal" lapse in memory is a natural part of aging and *not* necessarily indicative of the onset of AD. However, increased and abnormal worry about the possibility of developing the disease can be stressful and lead to the production of extra cortisol, which can be a contributing factor to advancing AD symptoms. Take proactive steps in order to mitigate your concerns; otherwise, you may create a self-fulfilling prophecy.

It *is* true, however, that, if someone in your family has AD, you're at a higher risk than the general population for developing the disease. In fact, for those who have a parent with AD, they are 3.5 times as likely to develop it, and the risk increases with each additional afflicted relative. In part, this genetic predisposition to the disease is due to the mutations of certain genes. However, this is *only one* of the risk factors, at least for late onset AD, which normally occurs after the age of 65.

According to the January 2012 *Archives of Neurology*, one of the best ways to limit your risk of developing AD is to stay cognitively active over your lifetime in order to prevent the accumulation of amyloids and to hinder the incidences of other pathology developing in the brain.

**"Whatever we expect with confidence
becomes our own self-fulfilling prophecy."**

~Brian Tracy

**"Alzheimer's is the cleverest thief,
because she not only steals from you,
but she steals the very thing you need
to remember what's been stolen."**

~Jarod Kintz
This Book Has No Title

U is for UNDERSTANDING

♦ **UNDERSTANDING: sympathetically aware of other people's feeling; tolerant and forgiving**

The words sympathy and empathy are often used interchangeably, but their meanings differ vastly.

While sympathy is the tendency to help others in order to prevent or alleviate their suffering without really understanding their plight, empathy is the ability to understand, perceive and share another person's feelings. When you are empathetic, you place yourself in the other person's position.

With these definitions in mind, you most likely are sympathetic to your parents' situation, but it is hard for you to imagine or truly feel the pain of their confusion since you have not experienced it yourself.

One of the hardest things to understand and accept about your interactions with your parents will be their tendency to repeat themselves. In fact, it's possible for you to have the same conversation twelve times in the short span of an hour. You repeat it gladly once or twice, especially if they are hard of hearing. By the time you get to the fourth or fifth time, you're ready to scream in frustration.

On one level, you're sympathetic and want to be patient and understanding.

On another level, you look to escape having the same conversation repeatedly. In the midst of these types of interactions, a good technique to practice is to mentally remove yourself from the situation by chanting the following mantra in your head.

"They do not remember what I just said.
Each time they listen to my words,
it's as if they are hearing them for the first time."

With this saying in mind, you can simply nod your head, repeat your words, and keep a pleasant demeanor as you answer the same questions time after time. This will do wonders to lessen your frustration.

"If there is any one secret of success,
it lies in the ability to get
the other person's point of view and see things
from that person's angle as well as from your own."
~Henry Ford

"Anger and intolerance are
the enemies of correct understanding."
~Mahatma Gandhi

is for *going on a* VOYAGE

♦ *going on a* VOYAGE: the act of taking a journey

Mourning the loss of a loved one is often referred to as *taking a journey through grief*. As your parents age, and especially when dementia is present, a "pre-journey" itinerary may also be set in motion.

Elisabeth Kübler-Ross, a pre-eminent thanatologist, in her book, *On Death and Dying*, contends that the grief journey involves five steps, which may or may not be addressed in the following order: (1) denial and isolation; (2) anger; (3) bargaining; (4) depression; and (5) acceptance. There's no need for concern, if you don't experience all of these phases. Think of this model as merely a framework that lets you know the emotions you are experiencing are universal; thus, feelings of isolation and/or the fear of "going crazy" with grief can be reduced.

Try to think of your grief over your parents' illness and the long, hard road in front of your family as a big brick wall that extends from the sky to the ground and spreads so wide that you can neither climb it nor go around it. The only healthy way to deal with your grief is to move right through it and experience all the pain (and surprising joy) you encounter along the way.

In truth, everything in life is a matter of attitude and perspective.

Consequently, while you are sad about your parents' decline, you may also be able to enjoy a simpler and more peaceful relationship with them than the type you might have experienced in prior years.

With a life stripped away to the bare bones, love is what most often remains. If possible, partake in the sweetness of the parent-child relationship, even if it is reversed at this point.

"Give sorrow words.
The grief that does not speak
whispers the o'erfraught heart and bids it break."

~William Shakespeare, Macbeth

"Death leaves a heartache no one can heal.
Love leaves a memory no one can steal."

~from a headstone in Ireland

"Even hundredfold grief is divisible by love."

~Terri Guillemets

is for WHAT'S THAT WORD?

♦ WHAT'S THAT WORD: difficulty in assigning the right word to an object, event or person

Language, a human brain function, is greatly affected by the onset of aging and dementia. Those with AD usually experience distinctive changes in their ability to word find and to remember names and places. Often there is difficulty in getting words out, usage of the wrong words, jumbling of words, misuse of proper grammatical structure, and a hesitation in speech.

If you're over 50, perhaps you've noticed that, at times, you have trouble finding the right word. It might only be a momentary lapse for you, but for your parents this is an everyday battle they fight. Just imagine how frightening it must be for them to lose the ability to name simple objects correctly.

Your parents might also have hearing issues which compound the language problem. Be on the lookout for the increasing use of phrases such as *I don't know* and *You know*. Additionally, instead of using the proper word or term, objects may be referred to as *that thing or whatchamaycallit* and people as *whatshername.*

Language function will continue to deteriorate over time. While your parents are still aware, they may continue to substitute a description for a lack of the proper word. When they become less aware, they may speak less often or not make sense. Additionally, the word "No" may increasingly become their *go-to* answer for any questioned posed.

It's so easy to become frustrated, especially when your parents "pretend" a problem with their language skills is nonexistent. In actuality, they're more frustrated than you, and probably a little embarrassed, as they struggle to get their thoughts out.

Keep in mind that fatigue further exacerbates their ability to communicate. Accordingly, don't start long or intense conversations late in the day, especially ones that might require a decision to be made.

It's also important to stay calm and exhibit patience throughout your conversations. If you exhibit agitation, they will mirror your emotions and simply be agitated further. Moreover, as hard as it might be to control your feelings, don't argue or tell your parents that they are wrong, even though you know they are mistaken. Those who reside in a demented state often get stuck in their own stories and these are the only truths they can comprehend.

In general, it may be wise to keep your conversations simple and/or ask easy-to-answer or yes/no questions.

**"I can remember
the frustration of not being able to talk.**

**I knew what I wanted to say,
but I could not get the words out,
so I would just scream."**

~Temple Grandin

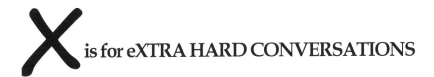

is for eXTRA HARD CONVERSATIONS

♦eXTRA HARD CONVERSATIONS:
talking about difficult or sensitive subjects

As your parents age and you begin to notice deviations in their behavior, there are many difficult conversations that you must have with them. One of the hardest talks will be about their driving capabilities and whether or not you should take away their car.

Simply said, a car equals freedom. After a lifetime of independence, it is unthinkable about how difficult it will be for your parents to relinquish their car keys along with their ability to live life on their own terms. Naturally, they rail against you when the topic is broached. However, beneath their bravado, they probably realize that it is becoming more difficult to concentrate while on the road.

Resolving this matter is not a one-time conversation. Instead, it must be discussed repeatedly with viable alternatives presented as to how they will be able to navigate the world going forward. As one alternative, many senior care communities include transportation services, and cities may offer special senior taxi services or buses.

Additional extra hard discussions may include the following.

1. Selling a cherished family home

2. Moving into an independent living or assisted living facility

3. Downsizing and disposing of beloved possessions due to lack of space

4. Transitioning to the use of a walker, wheelchair or scooter

5. Having a "minder" come in to provide companion care when necessary

6. Taking away access to their own finances

While it *is* important to evaluate the proper time to remove some of these responsibilities from your parents' plate, it helps to keep them involved in making as many decisions as they can. If you take away *all* of their responsibilities – because it's just easier for you to do it by yourself – you rob your parents of the opportunity to stretch their thinking and keep their brains active. Make sure to balance how much you do for them with allowing your parents to remain safely independent.

"When you have to make a choice and don't make it, that is in itself a choice."

~William James

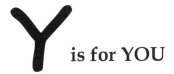

is for YOU

♦ YOU: the one being addressed

Caregiving is one of the hardest jobs you will ever have. It is not only physically taxing but mentally, emotionally and spiritually draining as well. Due to the enormous stress put on the caregiver's system, many are prone to burnout and clinical depression. This is why it is imperative to implement a program of self-care in order to regroup, refresh and rejuvenate.

Here are some tips on how to manage your situation.

1. *Don't be a martyr*. If you don't take care of yourself, you will not be able to take care of anyone else.

2. *Acknowledge your feelings*. There is no right or wrong way to feel – just the way you *do* feel. Repressing your mixed emotions about losing your own life vs. helping the parents you love only creates more stress and frustration. Look to create a safe environment where you can express your emotions openly with family members and friends. Additionally, don't beat yourself up for not doing enough. There is only so much effort you can expend that will actually help someone who lives in a demented state. Let go of guilt, for that is a useless emotion that accomplishes nothing. Instead, empower yourself by responding to your situation (thinking rationally and practically before acting) vs. reacting (acting emotionally without forethought).

3. ***Look for and accept support.*** Join a support group with people who are in the midst of a similar situation. Set up a schedule with friends and family members to relieve you of your duties so that you may have some downtime to relax.

4. ***Educate yourself.*** As Alzheimer's progresses, it is useful to be cognizant of what to expect so that you can be on the lookout for changes that herald the deepening of the demented state.

5. ***Avoid destructive behavior.*** Although you might wish to escape, indulging in alcohol, overeating and drug use will only exacerbate the situation and will result in having to deal with multiple problems. Moreover, it will be more difficult for you to handle your responsibilities because these behaviors play havoc with your health.

6. ***Be aware of community support.*** If you care for your parents at home, investigate in-home services, adult daycare and respite care services.

7. ***Eat right, exercise and get plenty of sleep.*** Exercise is a stress reducing activity, while proper nutrition fuels the body with energy so that you can complete tasks without fatigue. Additionally, a good night's sleep allows you to face a new day with a clear and rested mind so that you're able to function optimally.

8. ***Practice the art of positivity and adopt an attitude of gratitude.*** Changing your perspective to find the positive nugget in every situation affords a tremendous growth opportunity for you and allows you to reap the emotional rewards that come with caregiving for loved ones.

9. ***Practice meditation***. In silence and with controlled breathing, you can release your stress as you get in touch with your inner feelings and thoughts.

10. ***Smile and let laughter be your medicine***. Try to find the humor in your caregiving activities, even if it's laughing at the insanity of the situation. You may want to join a laughter club to relieve stress and bring a smile to your face. It's much easier to smile, which takes 17 muscles, than to frown, which takes 42. According to a Japanese proverb, *"one who smiles rather than rages is always the stronger."*

11. ***Carve out time for yourself***. Hold on to those activities you enjoy. Go to the movies; read a book; relax in the sun; play golf; or get together with friends. Although it may be difficult to schedule, do *not* let that deter you from their pursuit. It's important to retain a little bit of yourself when you are giving so much to another.

**"Don't sacrifice yourself too much,
because if you sacrifice too much,
there's nothing else you can give
and nobody will care for you."**

~Karl Lagerfeld

Z is for ZEN

♦ **ZEN: a school of thought that focuses on awareness through the practice of meditation**

When faced with issues of mortality, your parents *and* your own, you may look for comfort in religion, spirituality, or simply call upon your own inner strength as you search your soul in an attempt to unearth the answers to age-old questions about the meaning of life.

In truth, life is messy and can be an ostensibly endless list of tasks and responsibilities. At times, it may even seem as if you spend all your time jumping over the "puddles" of your life in order to land on a dry spot so you may have a moment to regroup before moving forward to, either, solve a new problem or seek happiness and further fulfillment.

While seeking happiness may be your goal, it is *not* a finite destination; rather, it is an attitude you hold as you travel along the road of life. In fact, the action of always seeking happiness indicates that you never feel happy because you're always in pursuit of the next thing that will make you feel that way. It's important to recognize, pause and relish the small moments of joy you encounter along your way. That is where true happiness resides.

Kathy Norris tells us that life *"in spite of the cost of living, is still popular!"*

The pursuit of the best life is made most worthwhile by the relationships you form and nurture. After all, that is the true meaning of life and why we exist; it is *to love and be loved.* The rest of life is spent taking care of the details.

At the time of your death, you will neither savor the wealth you've accumulated nor even laud your professional accomplishments. Your true wealth will be reflected by the loved ones who surround and support you as you let go of your physical body and move to what lies beyond.

As a caregiver, you have the opportunity to heap this sort of wealth upon your parents as you offer them the greatest gifts you have, which are love and care. And, perhaps, they may have lost their ability to communicate, but actions shout love louder than words ever could. Your parents will be cognizant of and revel in your final gifts to them.

"Happiness doesn't result from what we get, but from what we give."

~*Ben Carson*

"When it's all over, it's not who you were. It's whether you made a difference."

~*Bob Dole*

"For it is in giving that we receive."

~*St. Francis of Assisi*

BONUS SECTION:
43 INSPIRATIONAL TIPS FOR CAREGIVERS OF AGING PARENTS

If you are caring for an aging parent, or another loved one who suffers from Alzheimer's or another type of dementia, the following are some tips and thoughts on how to adjust your perspective and handle this situation with grace and a sense of humor.

As I'm sure you have noticed, I ended each section of this book with some words of wisdom from the philosophers of yesterday. In this section, I again utilize inspirational quotes.

I have always been a fan of quotes – and words in general. I first used them to inspire students when I taught high school English. They also inspire me to reflect and then write about what they mean to me.

I stand in awe of the beauty found in the sage words of others, and they bring me hope, a new level of awareness and an opportunity to consider a new perspective.

It's my fervent wish that you're enjoying and gleaning inspiration from the ones I've chosen to share with you.

TIP #1

Ronald Reagan said, *"You know, people get frustrated because their loved ones have Alzheimer's and say – 'Oh, he doesn't recognize me anymore.' 'How can I recognize this person, if they don't recognize me?' 'They're not the same person.' Well, they are the same person, but they've got a brain disease. And it's not their fault they've got this disease."*

A THOUGHT FOR CONSIDERATION

Anger is a manifestation of fear, and children caring for a parent with Alzheimer's can subconsciously fear many things. For example, that they may be genetically programmed for Alzheimer's; that they might have no one to care for them if and when the time comes when they're in need; or of their own mortality (if a parent dies, then they are "next up"). Before your fears are expressed as anger, delve below the surface and determine of what you are afraid.

TIP #2

Alexis Carrel said, *"All of us, at certain moments of our lives, need to take advice and to receive help from other people."*

A THOUGHT FOR CONSIDERATION

Taking care of an ill loved one can be a heavy burden, especially when you have to support him/her emotionally, physically and financially. If it's too overwhelming for you, don't be shy to ask for assistance or guidance from doctors, counselors, day care centers, relatives, friends or even your neighbors. When responsibilities and tasks are shared, they become more manageable and tend to lessen your isolation.

TIP #3

Amy Tan said: *"People think it's a terrible tragedy when somebody has Alzheimer's. But in my mother's case, it's different. My mother has been unhappy all her life. For the first time in her life, she's happy."*

A THOUGHT FOR CONSIDERATION

When a parent reverts to childlike behavior and the child becomes the parent, it's possible to repair rifts in relationships. Parents can return to a time of innocence before the slings and arrows of life hardened their heart and sent them spiraling down into a life of unhappiness and hurt, which, in turn, was afflicted upon their children. If you can let go of past hurts, you can enjoy the kinder, gentler and more child-like person who has emerged through Alzheimer's.

TIP #4

Gary Zukav said, *"Eventually you will come to understand that love heals everything, and love is all there is."*

A THOUGHT FOR CONSIDERATION

As you near the end of your days, fame and fortune won't matter much. It's only the people who surround you and the deep relationships you've nurtured throughout your life that will count. This is the meaning of life: to love and be loved.

Don't waste another moment: let your loved ones know how much they mean to you. Alzheimer's patients may have lost their ability to communicate with words, but they still understand loving touch and actions ... even if it's just in the moment.

TIP #5

Ralph Waldo Emerson said, *"When it is dark enough, you can see the stars."*

A THOUGHT FOR CONSIDERATION

Life is lived in the contrast between the spectrum of light and dark; good and bad, positive and negative, etc. These circumstances reflect the natural duality of the world. Experiencing both ends allows you to better understand and appreciate each situation in which you find yourself. Thus, caregiving can be regarded as both a burden AND a blessing. It all depends where you stand on the continuum of duality and which way you choose to look.

TIP #6

Stephen R. Covey said, *"Opposition is a natural part of life. Just as we develop our physical muscles through overcoming opposition such as lifting weights, we develop our character muscles by overcoming challenges and adversity."*

A THOUGHT FOR CONSIDERATION

Although caregiving is wrought with difficulties, you are learning life lessons that can serve you well for the rest of your days. To name a few – you're developing patience, an empathetic nature, and a full appreciation of the littlest moments/triumphs of life. Remember these lessons and put them into action in all aspects of your life – not just when it comes to caregiving. You will be happier for it.

TIP #7

Zig Ziglar said, *"You cannot tailor make your situation in life, but you can tailor make your attitudes to fit those situations."*

A THOUGHT FOR CONSIDERATION

Your contentment with your life circumstances all comes down to your attitude towards them. You can either say, *"Oh no! Another problem to solve!"* OR *"Oh goody! Another problem I CAN solve!"* Just think of how empowered you will feel when you're able to figure out a solution that can be of benefit to both you and your loved one for whom you are caring.

TIP #8

Sir James M. Barrie said, *"Those who bring sunshine into the lives of others cannot keep it from themselves."*

A THOUGHT FOR CONSIDERATION

The world is a giant mirror. Therefore, whatever thoughts and actions you emit into the universe, they are reflected back into your life.

For example, if you're feeling frustrated with your situation, you will most probably be met by more circumstances that will increase your frustration. Conversely, if you approach your caregiving duties with patience, your loved ones will also exhibit a calm and even demeanor.

TIP #9

Rikki Rogers said, *"Strength doesn't come from what you can do. It comes from overcoming the things you once thought you couldn't."*

A THOUGHT FOR CONSIDERATION

Caregiving stretches your emotional muscles – sometimes more than you ever thought possible. It's a lot like exercise; you don't really want to do it, but you are rewarded, IF you can power through your resistance and achiness. In turn, this empowers you to reach deeper within your wellspring of strength in order to help your loved ones travel the difficult roads of Alzheimer's.

TIP #10

A physician once said, *"The best medicine for humans is love."* Someone asked, *"What if it doesn't work?"* He smiled and said, *"Increase the dose."*

A THOUGHT FOR CONSIDERATION

Although there are some prescribed medications for dementia, such as *Namenda* and *Aricept*, ultimately, there is no cure. In some cases, these only delay the inevitable symptoms.

Truly, the "spoonful of sugar" that makes this bitter pill of a disease go down (or be manageable) is love mixed with a big dose of respect, honor and empathy.

TIP #11

In *The Wedding*, Nicholas Sparks wrote: *"Every time I read to her, it was like I was courting her, because sometimes, just sometimes, she would fall in love with me again, just like she had a long time ago. And that's the most wonderful feeling in the world. How many people are ever given that chance? To have someone you love fall in love with you over and over?"*

A THOUGHT FOR CONSIDERATION

Sparks describes the essence of my most favorite concept: the *"do-over."* Here's how it applies to caregiving. It's easy to get upset while offering care to a loved one, and, accordingly, you might lash out in anger or frustration at him or her. However, on the bright side, he/she will most likely forget the incident. This allows you to do better each day. In a nutshell, you get to have multiple do-overs until you learn to strike the best emotional balance with your loved one.

TIP #12

Helen Keller said, *"The world is full of suffering, and it is also full of overcoming it."*

A THOUGHT FOR CONSIDERATION

When you're able to address the loss of a parent, AND figure out how to move through this circumstance in a healthy manner, you might consider turning around to help the next person who is approaching this difficult time in his/her life. I imagine that if everyone would put his/her hand out to help another, we could all end up holding hands. This certainly would make burdens easier to carry.

TIP #13

Carol Bowlby Sifton, BScOT, founding editor of *Alzheimer's Care Quarterly* wrote: *"All of a sudden, the person (with Alzheimer's) might not eat, but it's not because he or she is being difficult on purpose."*

A THOUGHT FOR CONSIDERATION

Those with dementia aren't trying to be difficult when they refuse to eat. They might be confused or embarrassed because they have forgotten how to use a utensil. Additionally, eating is usually a time for social interaction, so they might feel at a loss to participate and, thus, withdraw from the activity.

My mother chews her food and then spits most of it out. I'm at a loss to figure out why she does this. Perhaps, it's because once the flavor is gone, she feels there's no reason to swallow. Since a person's swallowing mechanism is often affected by Alzheimer's, another reason could be that she's afraid of choking if she swallows the chewed up food. You might also want to check if your loved one has ill-fitting dentures, cuts or sores on the mouth, or eye issues which could alter depth perception and/or focus so that he/she has difficulty seeing the food/plate and raising a utensil to the mouth.

My mother has also forgotten her likes/dislikes and needs to be reminded. With prompting and serving her bite-size and easily chewable portions, she'll try an item. Of course, ice cream is exempted. She will ALWAYS eat ice cream, and it goes down with such ease.

TIP #13 *continued*

To make sure she is receiving enough nutritional value, if she doesn't eat much at a meal, I supplement with a can of Ensure Plus.

To people who don't have a disorder of the brain, eating is a simple procedure. To a person with Alzheimer's, the task can be overwhelming. In fact, if at your next meal you consciously think about how many steps you mindlessly take when eating, you will have more of an appreciation of its complexity.

TIP #14

Most everyone has heard the old adage, *"When life gives you lemons, make lemonade!"*

A THOUGHT FOR CONSIDERATION

Some days never start out the way you want them to, but that doesn't mean you can't turn it around. Even the bad moments won't last forever.

Remain optimistic and face the "bad" with the intention to find the nugget of good in each situation. Try not to lose sight of the positivity which surrounds you every day – IF you choose to look for it. Use it to stay focused and allow it to help you release your inner smile. Smiling creates a clear path directly to the heart of another.

TIP #15

Every day, you get to make a conscious decision to either *be a PENCIL, which can help to write/create happy moments* OR *an ERASER, which can help to alleviate sadness.*

A THOUGHT FOR CONSIDERATION

No matter which alternative you choose, your caregiving gives you the power to change a person's life – even if it's only for a few seconds out of a day.

TIP #16

Cheryl Richardson said, *"When we think good thoughts, we feel good. When we feel good, we make good choices. When we feel good and make good choices, we draw more good experiences into our lives. It really is that simple ... and elegant ... and true."*

A THOUGHT FOR CONSIDERATION

Words such as good and nice seem like very benign ones, and they can pale in the face of superlatives such as fantastic, terrific or the best. However, there is power in simplicity and just being plain old good or nice.

In fact, think about the power of the word "good" in the following statement by Cavett Robert: *"If you don't think every day is a good day, just try missing one."*

TIP #17

Hugh Black wrote: *"The duty of happiness becomes clearer when we see how it affects others. A sunny soul brings sunshine everywhere. It is the merry heart that makes the cheerful countenance, and it is the cheerful countenance that spreads cheer to make other hearts merry. A bright and happy temperament is a great social asset, adding to the happiness of the world."*

A THOUGHT FOR CONSIDERATION

Accordingly, each day, try to bring a little bit of sunshine into the life of the person for whom you are caregiving. It will make a difference in both of your lives!

TIP #18

Are you feeling sort of down and wearing a frown? Don't worry! You haven't lost your smile. It's right under your nose. You just forgot it was there!

A THOUGHT FOR CONSIDERATION

It's easy to get caught up in negativity when you are observing your loved one slipping away from you a little bit more each day. It's important to *consciously remind yourself* to rediscover your sense of gratitude, as well as your smile. This can be accomplished by thinking about all the things and people you *do* have in your life. See if you can elicit a smile from your loved one. It can light up the moment, and it's in these moments where we all live and love.

TIP #19

Jim Rohn said, *"One person caring about another represents life's greatest value."*

A THOUGHT FOR CONSIDERATION

Caring and caregiving are two ways to reap that value. Although very difficult at times, the rewards are also great. Volunteering at my mom's assisted living facility and bestowing simple kindnesses on the residents (and seeing their gratitude) fills my heart with warmth knowing that I was able to help a fellow human being.

TIP #20

Kurt Vonnegut said, *"Laughter and tears are both responses to frustration and exhaustion. I myself prefer to laugh, since there is less cleaning up to do afterward."*

A THOUGHT FOR CONSIDERATION

It's important to try to keep a sense of humor about your caregiving duties and the sometimes absurd situations that need addressing. Laughter really is the best medicine and the strongest type you can take to strengthen your body and mind. It relaxes the whole body; it boosts the immune system; it triggers the release of endorphins and lowers stress hormones; decreases pain; prevents heart disease; improves mood; and eases anxiety and fear.

That's one medicine which I wouldn't mind taking!

TIP #21

Lena Horne said, *"It's not the load that breaks you down, it's the way you carry it."*

A THOUGHT FOR CONSIDERATION

When it comes to caregiving (and most situations in life), it's your attitude that matters most. Don't be a martyr and feel obligated to handle your caregiving duties on your own. There's support to be had. You just have to look for it, and, when offered, accept it. Think of your gracious receipt of help as a gift to the giver, for he/she gets to feel good about helping. In truth, giving and receiving are two sides of the same coin.

TIP #22

Michael Scott said, *"You must learn to heed your senses. Humans use but a tiny percentage of theirs. They barely look, they rarely listen, they never smell, and they think that they can only experience feelings through their skin. But they talk, oh, do they talk."*

A THOUGHT FOR CONSIDERATION

Communication takes on a new flavor and challenge when those with Alzheimer's have difficulty with proper word finding. Accordingly, when you address this person, speak in short sentences and use visual clues. Also, learn to communicate with all the senses. For example, show love by sharing a warm hug; providing comfort food or a sweet treat; stirring memories with strong and familiar fragrances; singing familiar songs; or reminiscing with family photographs.

TIP #23

Polly Berrien Berends said, *"Everything that happens to you is your teacher. The secret is to learn to sit at the feet of your own life and be taught by it. Everything that happens is either a blessing, which is also a lesson, OR a lesson, which is also a blessing."*

A THOUGHT FOR CONSIDERATION

Your contentment with your particular set of circumstances all rests in your perception of it and your attitude towards it. You can choose to view your caregiving duties as a burden that wears you down OR as a blessing for which you're able to reap the rewards.

TIP #24

Bryant McGill said, *"Every soul is beautiful and precious; it is worthy of dignity and respect and deserving of peace, joy and love."*

A THOUGHT FOR CONSIDERATION

Your loved one still lives inside his/her body and mind, even though both have probably deteriorated from Alzheimer's and/or another affliction. Accordingly, refrain from talking negatively about him/her to others as if he/she can't hear or understand you. Even if all the words are not fully comprehended, body language and tone speak volumes. Honor your loved one by always being respectful of his/her feelings.

TIP #25

In the movie, *Network,* one of the characters says: *"Stand up wherever you are, go to the nearest window and yell as loud as you can: 'I'm mad as hell, and I'm not going to take it anymore.'"*

A THOUGHT FOR CONSIDERATION

As a caregiver, do you ever feel like yelling out the window like the character in the movie? It CAN be a beneficial exercise, although I suggest you think of it more as a metaphor. You don't have to shout from a real window, but only from the "window" of your soul. It's natural to be angry about the suffering of a loved one and frustrated with the situation. Express your feelings appropriately and expel them from your body. This can clear your mind so you can turn to more proactive thoughts and actions.

TIP #26

Nothing is new, until it happens to you. That's the difference between empathy and sympathy.

A THOUGHT FOR CONSIDERATION

Sympathy is essentially feeling sorry for someone and wishing he would feel better. It may also include a value judgment. Conversely, empathy is the actual understanding of the situation of another because you have the ability to put yourself in his shoes. This is most often accomplished by those who have experienced something similar because they "get it" – as you do now. Developing an empathetic nature, which is of true help to others in need, is one of the blessings of caregiving for an ill loved one.

TIP #27

How can you come to understand duality? *It's all in the contrast.*

A THOUGHT FOR CONSIDERATION

Caregiving for an aging parent reflects the natural duality of the world. You get to experience both ends of the spectrum of life as your parents revert to childlike behavior due to illness and you become the parental figure for them. When you're frustrated by their inability to complete easy (for you) tasks, try to recall the patience your parent had when you were a child and you inundated them with incessant questions or expressed the desire to hear the same books read multiple times.

TIP #28

Martin Luther King, Jr. said, *"We must accept finite disappointment, but we must never lose infinite hope."*

A THOUGHT FOR CONSIDERATION

While it's true that Alzheimer's and other dementias all follow the same path to deterioration and demise, it's also true that you can keep hope alive in the moments you spend with your loved ones. You can ignite these sparks of hope by eliciting a smile or a chuckle; with a warm embrace; with a show of respect; with a helping hand; and simply by showing up. Life is lived in the moments when we connect with those for whom we care deeply.

TIP #29

A.A. Milne wrote, *"Promise me you'll always remember: You're braver than you believe, and stronger than you seem, and smarter than you think."*

A THOUGHT FOR CONSIDERATION

As caring, loving and supportive as you are of the person for whom you're caregiving, you are also a human being who has human failings. Thus, sometimes, you'll get frustrated and not handle a situation as well as you could have. Don't beat yourself up about it; you'll do better next time. Instead, take a breath and appreciate all the days that you've been at the top of your game. You're doing a great job! Pat yourself on the shoulder.

TIP #30

Abraham Lincoln said, *"With the fearful strain that is on me night and day, if I did not laugh, I should die."*

A THOUGHT FOR CONSIDERATION

Although Abe Lincoln was talking about a dire issue that affected an entire nation, to you, your caregiving duties may be at the center of your universe. Caregiver relief comes in various ways, and laughter is one great way to decrease tension. Take the time to watch a funny movie, read a funny book, attend a comedy show or participate in any activity that allows you to release great big belly laughs.

TIP #31

Jonathan Anthony Burkett said, *"For a permanent solution to easing tension and soothing the rough waters of the world that cause people to go to drugs, drinking … overeating, or anything that will give them some temporary relief, you can't beat the support and encouragement of a friend."*

A THOUGHT FOR CONSIDERATION

Avoid self-medicating to relieve the pressure of your caregiving duties. No one is a mind reader. If you need help and support, make sure to ask for it and be specific about what types of things would assist you the most. Most people want to offer assistance; they are just at a loss to imagine what that would entail. Help them out and make a list!!

TIP #32

Theodore N. Vail said, *"Real difficulties can be overcome; it is only the imaginary ones that are unconquerable."*

A THOUGHT FOR CONSIDERATION

Those with Alzheimer's often have many fears brought on by paranoia. Since they have lost their ability to think logically, your reasonable explanation will most likely fall on deaf ears. Instead, try distracting the person by changing the conversation, or, without agreeing with the issue, tell him/her that you will investigate the problem and report back what you discover. Whether or not the situation can be remedied, simply knowing someone is looking out for him/her will have a calming effect. Everyone feels better when their feelings are validated.

TIP #33

Elbert Hubbard said, *"The greatest mistake a man can ever make is to be afraid of making one."* He also said, *"There is no failure except in no longer trying."*

A THOUGHT FOR CONSIDERATION

Any caregiver can make a mistake, get frustrated, or "lose it" momentarily from the stress of the situation. That's ok; you're human, and these are natural reactions to a situation in which you're not really sure what is the most helpful and what actions can make your loved one more comfortable and less fearful.

Trying your best is all you can ask of yourself. Remember, with a little "tri" you can become tri-umphant!

TIP #34

Jim Valvano said, *"If you laugh, you think, and you cry, that's a full day. That's a heck of a day. You do that seven days a week, you're going to have something special."*

A THOUGHT FOR CONSIDERATION

To experience a good day with your loved one, you don't have to make very elaborate or complicated plans. In fact, the simpler the better. Get back to basics by simply showing up, and this alone can make that day special for you and your loved one.

TIP #35

It's often said that as a person ages, he/she enters his/her *golden years*. I don't know … are they really golden? Maybe, they should be categorized as their *wonder years*?

A THOUGHT FOR CONSIDERATION

Here's what I mean by that comment. As the populace ages, people can start to wonder some of the following: *I wonder where my keys are; I wonder where my purse went; I wonder where I live; I wonder who you are; I wonder what year this is*, and so on.

Before the "wondering" reaches this point, ask your loved one to help you locate and secure important documents (wills, insurance policies, deeds, etc.), as well as record for safekeeping bank, household and any other important information.

I'm in the midst of preparing a soft-cover book that will help you to record all these kinds of pertinent information – for yourself as well as your parents. Upon completion, if you get the information that you've transcribed into the book notarized, it can become part of your estate planning.

For further information on the publication date, please contact me at LNGerst@LNGerst.com.

"I have so much paperwork,
I'm afraid my paperwork has paperwork."

~Gabrielle Zevin~
Elsewhere

TIP #36

Amy Bloom said, *"You are imperfect, permanently and inevitably flawed. And you are beautiful."*

A THOUGHT FOR CONSIDERATION

You may look at the people for whom you are caring as broken because they are not as they once were. However, they're not imperfect, but perfect because of their imperfections. In fact, we're all broken in our own ways AND all beautiful because of it. The aged and diseased are simply transformed into a new kind of beautiful creature who we must learn to honor.

TIP #37

What would happen if you realized how powerful you really are?

A THOUGHT FOR CONSIDERATION

As you watch your loved one slip away – and you know that you're unable to halt this progression – it's easy to feel disempowered by your lack of options. However, there is something powerful you CAN do. In your hands, you hold the ability to bring moments of light to a person who lives in an often dark and confusing place. And that's a very powerful thing!

TIP #38

In *The Wizard of Oz*, the Tin Man said, *"Hearts will never be practical until they are unbreakable."*

A THOUGHT FOR CONSIDERATION

One reason why it pains you to see your loved one suffering is because you feel great love for him or her. And, there's no getting around it – when we love, there's always the risk of loss. Ask yourself, *"Would I give up the wonderful past I've shared with my loved one in order to escape the current hard work of caregiving?"* I'm betting the answer is, *"Probably not."*

TIP #39

Francis Bacon wrote, *"A sudden bold and unexpected question doth many times surprise a man and lay him open."*

A THOUGHT FOR CONSIDERATION

When a parent or another loved one becomes ill, it forces you to confront fears and issues that you might have been avoiding, for example, your own health.

Use this opportunity and time wisely by taking better care of yourself, getting more sleep, and reducing stress. Furthermore, make sure to communicate your feelings of love and devotion to your friends and family. Don't *ass-u-me* that they know how you feel about them.

Tip #40

Thema Davis said, *"Don't be afraid to sit in respectful silence with the bereaved."*

A Thought For Consideration

When someone is going through a storm, your silent presence is more powerful than a million empty words. When your loved one no longer has the capacity to communicate with words, a loving and supportive silence can still telegraph love, respect and devotion.

Tip #41

Erma Bombeck said the *definition of guilt is the gift that keeps on giving.*

A Thought For Consideration

Caregivers tend to be hard on themselves, thinking they're not doing enough and then feeling guilty about it. When you beat yourself up about things you might/might not have said and done in the past, AND you're unrelenting in your berating, you're actually abusing yourself. You can't change the past, but you certainly have the power to do better in the present and future. Save your energy for this *vs.* draining it with the useless emotions of guilt and regret.

Tip #42

Elizabeth Bowen said, *"If you look at life one way, there is always cause for alarm."*

A THOUGHT FOR CONSIDERATION

Your attitude makes all the difference. Try looking at the world through *eyes of love* (not romantically but with compassion and kindness) *vs.* through the *eyes of fear*, which encourages you to act out because you don't know what the future holds and this fact frightens you.

Tip #43

Ursula K. LeGuin said, *"If you see a whole thing - it seems that it's always beautiful. Planets, lives... But up close a world's all dirt and rocks. And day to day, life's a hard job; you get tired; you lose the pattern."*

A THOUGHT FOR CONSIDERATION

Make sure to afford yourself the time to step back from your life and the minutia of your caregiving duties. This will allow you to see the big picture and remember WHY you've decided to take on a caregiving role and the difference it's making in the life of your loved one.

EXCERPT #1 FROM

"A GUIDE FOR CAREGIVERS OF AGING PARENTS WITH ALZHEIMER'S: WORDS OF ASSISTANCE, COMFORT & SUPPORT"

YOU ARE NOT ALONE

As I mentioned in the previous section, loss can be very isolating. However, I want you to know that you're NOT alone – *even when it feels that way.*

Emerging feelings of isolation are often *self-imposed* because many have a tendency to push people away when they're hurting. They may feel like a burden to others, if they appear to be weak and in need of help.

The truth is that this is the time when you require a support network the most, and friends and family are usually more than willing to reach out a helping hand. The rest is up to you because you need to *allow yourself to accept* the offered help. Keep in mind that it's your relationships with others that will provide the most assistance in coping with your situation.

When you keep all your emotions to yourself – tempered down and bottled up inside – you can become a volcano that can literally explode at any moment. It's beneficial to air your feelings because they may sound different and less overwhelming when expressed aloud *vs.* having them only roll around in your brain. I call this the *bounce back effect*, which provides a reality check and allows you to receive feedback from others who can help you to see possible resolutions to your issues.

The enormity of the task in front of you can seem overwhelming, and you may not even know where to begin. Some of the best ways to learn about what this undertaking is going to entail include: completing your due diligence on caregiving and the types of dementia, especially Alzheimer's Disease; talking to professionals; and communing in a support group with those in similar situations.

Remember, along with your feelings of isolation and fear, your loved one is also feeling isolated and scared. And, it's probably going to be your job to allay these frightening emotions that can compound the effects of the disease.

Once your parent or other loved one has started the march towards dependence on you and others, it's a journey where there's no turning back. Even if they are in a stage where they're not totally aware of what's going on, they still probably know that a move out their own home means that they're relinquishing their independence, which they know will never be recaptured. The uncertainty of what comes next in this scenario is a breeding ground for fear and agitated emotions.

Thus, for a smoother transition from independence to dependency, and in order to temper isolating and confusing feelings, start each day with a pledge to your parents that you are there to support them through all of these changes and you will ensure their safety. If they are able to maintain a calm demeanor, this will allow you to remain calm, too.

EXCERPT #2 FROM

"A GUIDE FOR CAREGIVERS OF AGING PARENTS WITH ALZHEIMER'S: WORDS OF ASSISTANCE, COMFORT & SUPPORT"

SPRING ALWAYS FOLLOWS WINTER

Due to your circumstances, you may feel as if you're living in the winter of your discontent. The gloomy prognosis that has been delivered, along with your ever-increasing caretaking role, can certainly make it seem pretty cold and dark. If you're feeling this way, I suggest that you take a page from nature's script, which says: *"No matter how long the winter, spring is sure to follow."*

When you're coping with the many medical issues of your parents, it's easy to get stuck in a space that feels cold, dark and wintery. You "bundle up" to protect yourself from outside forces that make you sad or are too hurtful in which to participate.

Try to recall the feelings you might have on the first day of Spring, which is a great time to take a positive step forward for it is heralded as a glorious time of rebirth and renewal.

Harriet Ann Jacobs said the following:

> *"The beautiful spring came; and when Nature resumes her loveliness, the human soul is apt to revive also."*

During this season, as it gets warmer outside, you naturally begin to shed your winter layers of clothing.

Please consider the idea of figuratively doing the same with those feelings and behaviors that are preventing you from coping and healing.

As you continue down your path of caregiving, I ask you to continue to shed more of the layers you've worn in your winter of discontent, which may include anger, resentment or fear. If you can rid yourself of some of that extra weight, the sunshine of life will be better able to penetrate the depths of your soul.

"In the depth of winter, I finally learned that there was in me an invincible summer."

~Albert Camus~

"Hope is the only bee that makes honey without flowers."

~Robert Green Ingersoll~

"I go to nature to be soothed and healed and to have my senses put in order."

~John Burroughs~

To read more, you can purchase *"A Guide for Caregivers of Aging Parents with Alzheimer's: Words of Assistance, Comfort and Inspiration"* at the following link.

http://www.amazon.com/Guide-Caregivers-Aging-Parents-Alzheimers/dp/1494402408

AUTHOR BIO

Ellen Gerst is a Grief and Relationship Coach, an author and a workshop leader who helps her clients and readers to experience a change in perspective so that they're able to move gracefully through difficult life circumstances. In turn, this allows them to find success and a renewal of their zest for living and loving.

She is the author of several books on grief and relationships, as well as topics that include: spirituality, caregiving for aging parents, networking and social media for entrepreneurs, building confidence and the importance of a positive attitude.

Titles include: *Suddenly Single: How To Find Renewal After Loss; 101 Tips and Thoughts on Coping with Grief; 52 Secrets on How You Can Cope With Your Grief; How To Mourn: Help For Those Who Grieve and the Ones Who Help Them; Words of Comfort To Pave Your Journey of Loss; Love After Loss: Writing The Rest of Your Story; 52 Secrets for a Successful Relationship; If You Want To Be Terrific, You Need To Be Specific; Available Choices for Dating After 35+; Figuring Out Life and Death: Musings, Stories and Questions About Suicide; 52 Reasons To Smile; Lighten Up and Smile: The Power of Positive Thoughts; Mastering The Art of Intimate Relationships;* and *A Guide for Caregivers of Aging Parents with Alzheimer's: Words of Assistance, Comfort and Inspiration.*

Title from her A to Z series include: *Understanding Dating & Relationships From A to Z; Understanding Grief from A to Z; Understanding Spirituality from A to Z; Understanding Fitness & Weight Loss From A to Z;* and *Understanding Networking & Social Media for Entrepreneurs From A to Z.*

Contact Information

Connect with Ellen and find out more about her products and services via her websites.

1. Main Website Dedicated to Grief and Relationships
   http://www.LNGerst.com

2. Website Dedicated to Spirituality
   http://www.UnderstandingSpiritualityFromAtoZ.blogspot.com

3. Website Dedicated to Caregiving
   http://www.CaregivingForAgingParents.blogspot.com

4. Connect on Facebook for dating and relationship tips
   http://www.facebook.com/FindingLoveAfterLoss

5. Connect on Facebook for coping with grief tips
   http://www.facebook.com/WordsOfComfortToPaveYourJourneyOfLoss

6. Connect on Pinterest for coping with caregiving tips
   http://www.pinterest.com/ellengerst/help-with-caregiving-for-those-with-alzheimers/

7. Find Books on Amazon
   http://amzn.to/w27mnt

8. Find Books on Barnes and Noble
   http://bit.ly/LK5SJz

Other Resources

1. Meditation Made Easy
   http://www.UnderstandingSpiritualityFromAtoZ.blogspot.com/p/meditation-made-easy.html

2. Free E-book: Coping with Grief Tips & Thoughts
   http://www.lngerst.com/Coping_With_Grief_Resources.html#Coping_with_Grief

Printed in Poland
by Amazon Fulfillment
Poland Sp. z o.o., Wrocław